I Care About
MY BODY

Liz Lennon

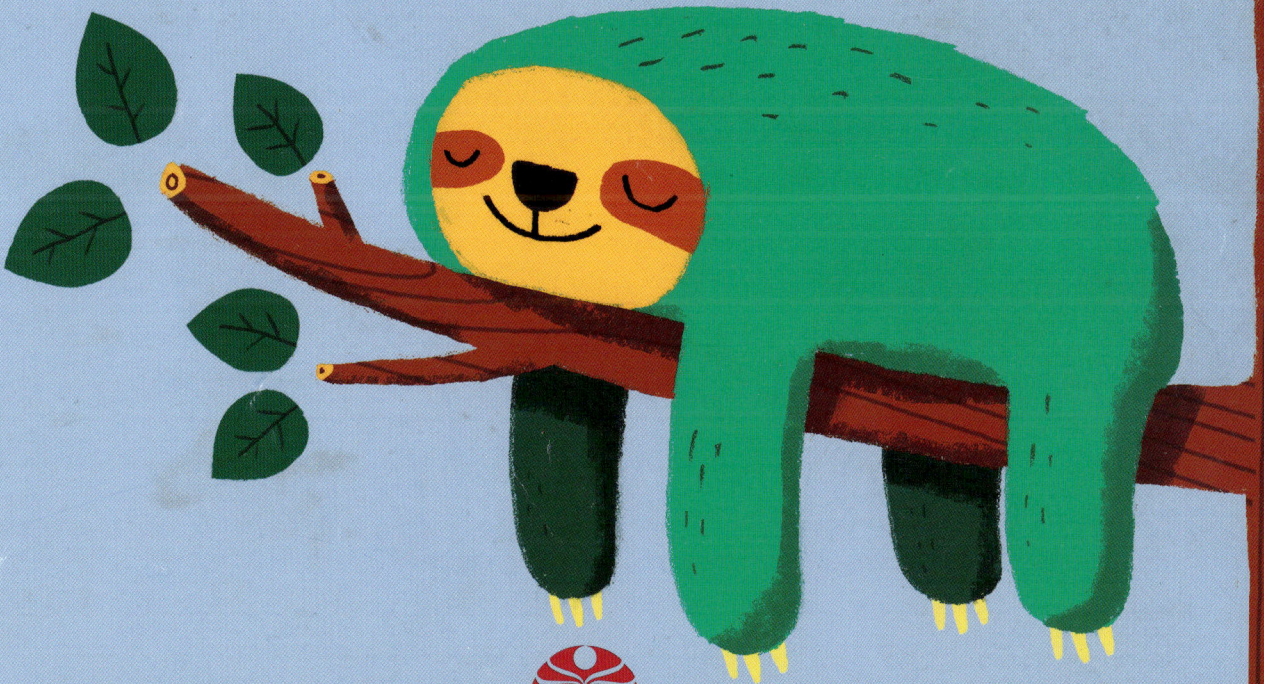

CRABTREE
PUBLISHING COMPANY
WWW.CRABTREEBOOKS.COM

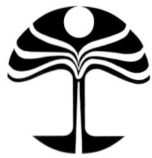

CRABTREE
PUBLISHING COMPANY
WWW.CRABTREEBOOKS.COM

Published in Canada
Crabtree Publishing
616 Welland Avenue
St. Catharines, ON
L2M 5V6

Published in the United States
Crabtree Publishing
347 Fifth Ave,
Suite 1402-145
New York, NY 10016

Published by Crabtree Publishing Company in 2021

First published in 2020 by The Watts Publishing Group
Copyright © The Watts Publishing Group, 2020

Printed in the U.S.A./122020/CG20201014

Author: Liz Lennon

Editorial director: Kathy Middleton

Editors: Sarah Peutrill, Janine Deschenes

Design: Collaborate

Illustrator: Michael Buxton

Proofreader: Melissa Boyce

Production coordinator
 & Prepress technician: Samara Parent

Print coordinator: Katherine Berti

Library and Archives Canada Cataloguing in Publication

Title: I care about my body / Liz Lennon.
Other titles: My body
Names: Lennon, Liz (Children's non-fiction writer), author. | Buxton, Michael (Artist), illustrator.
Description: Illustrated by Michael Buxton. |
 Previously published: London: Franklin Watts, 2020. | Includes index.
Identifiers: Canadiana (print) 20200357794 | Canadiana (ebook) 20200357859 |
 ISBN 9781427128904 (hardcover) |
 ISBN 9781427128966 (softcover) |
 ISBN 9781427129024 (HTML)
Subjects: LCSH: Health—Juvenile literature. | LCSH: Hygiene—Juvenile literature.
Classification: LCC RA777 .L46 2021 | DDC j613—dc23

Library of Congress Cataloging-in-Publication Data

Names: Lennon, Liz (Children's non-fiction writer) author. | Buxton, Michael, illustrator.
Title: I care about my body / Liz Lennon ; illustrated by Michael Buxton.
Description: New York, NY : Crabtree Publishing Company, 2021. |
 Series: I care about | Includes index.
Identifiers: LCCN 2020045665 (print) | LCCN 2020045666 (ebook) |
 ISBN 9781427128904 (hardcover) |
 ISBN 9781427128966 (paperback) |
 ISBN 9781427129024 (ebook)
Subjects: LCSH: Hygiene--Juvenile literature. | Health--Juvenile literature.
Classification: LCC RA777 .L46 2021 (print) | LCC RA777 (ebook) |
 DDC 613--dc23
LC record available at https://lccn.loc.gov/2020045665
LC ebook record available at https://lccn.loc.gov/2020045666

Contents

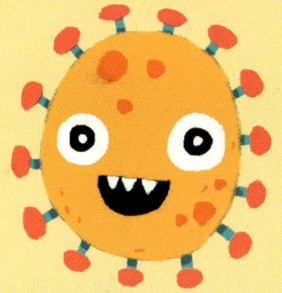

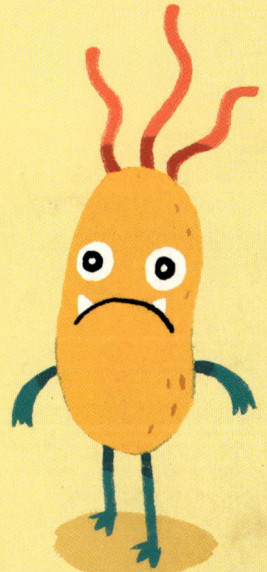

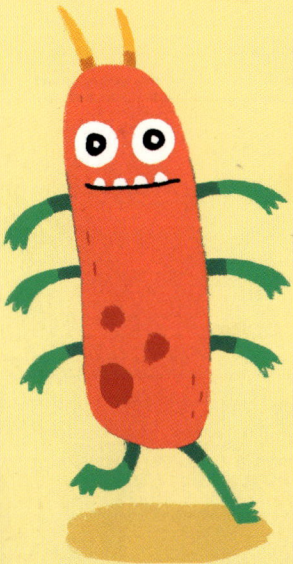

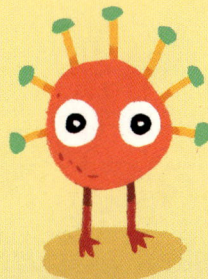

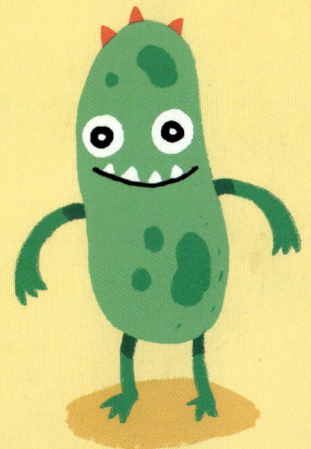

Your brilliant body

Your body is amazing. Under your skin there are **muscles** and bones that help you move and **organs** that keep you alive. Your heart pumps blood around your body. Your lungs let you breathe. Your brain makes sure everything works as it should.

You can do so many things with your body. You can read this page. You can play games and have fun. Your body is amazing—but it is important to take care of it. Find out in this book how you can care for your body.

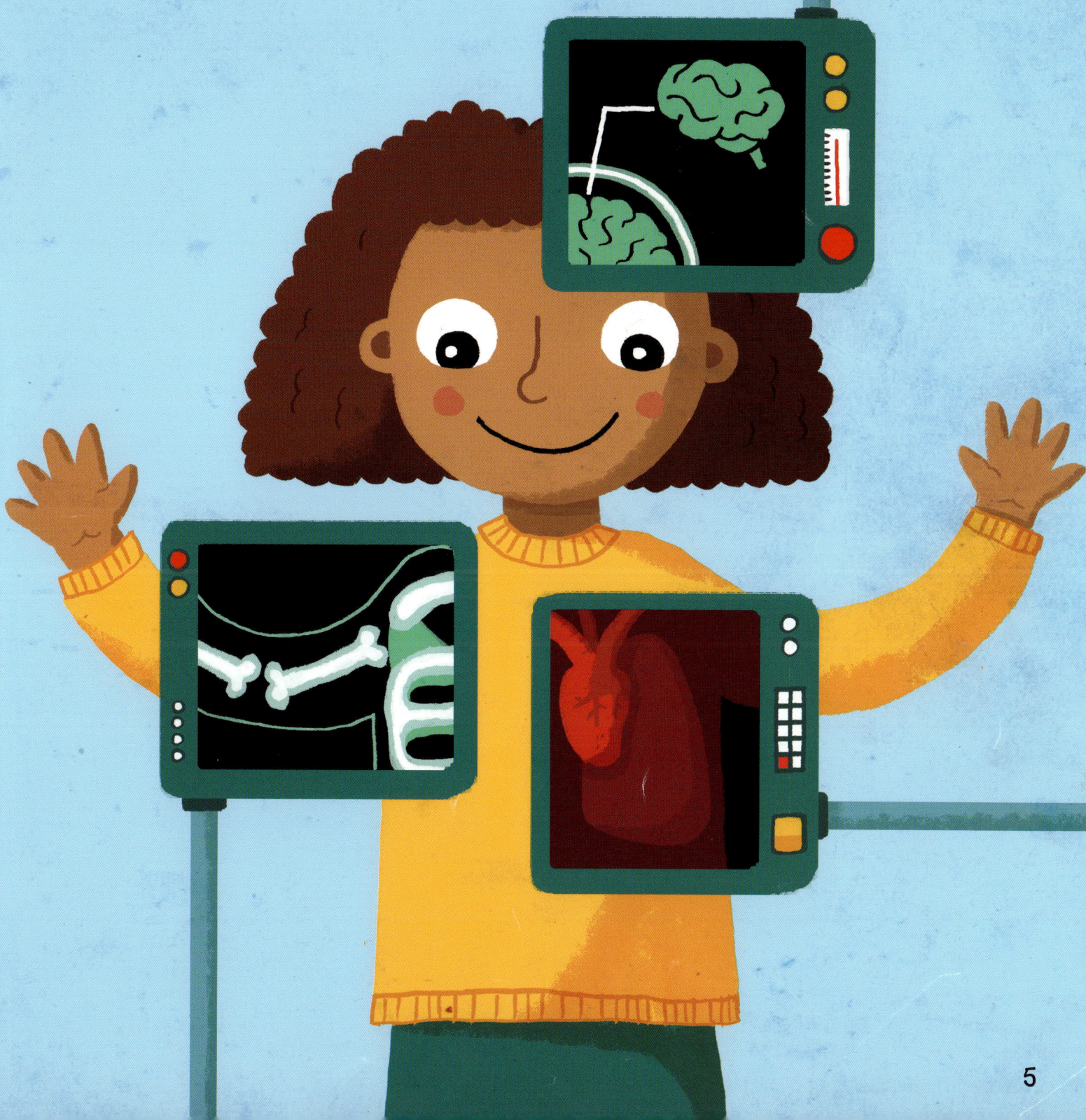

What should I eat?

Food helps your body in different ways. Some foods, such as bananas and eggs, give your body a lot of **energy**. Other foods, such as green vegetables, help make your teeth and bones strong. Eating different kinds of healthy foods is an important way to keep your body healthy.

Look on the next page to see some examples of healthy foods.

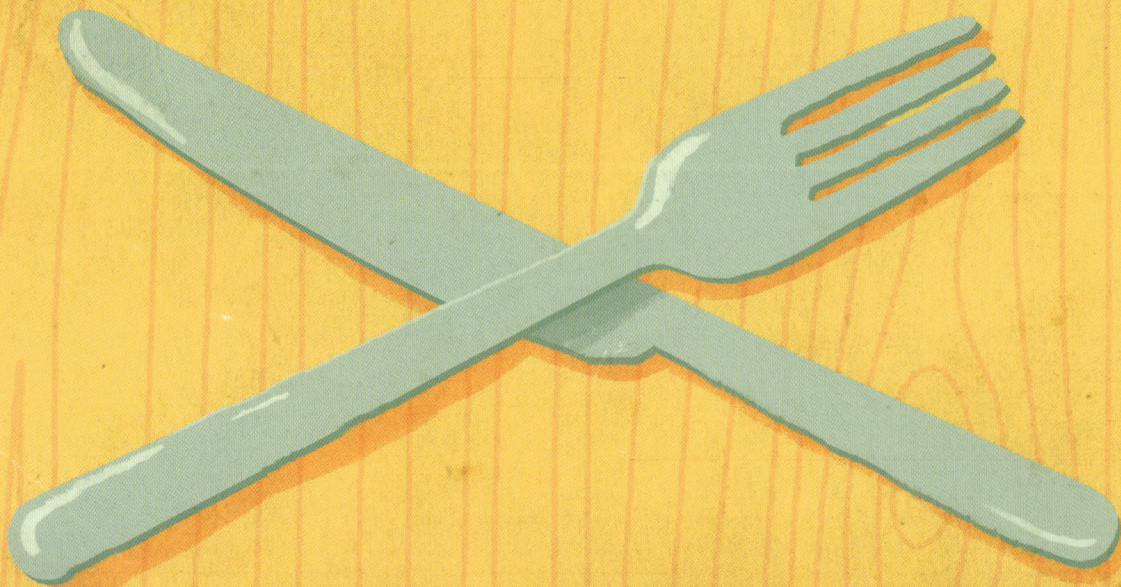

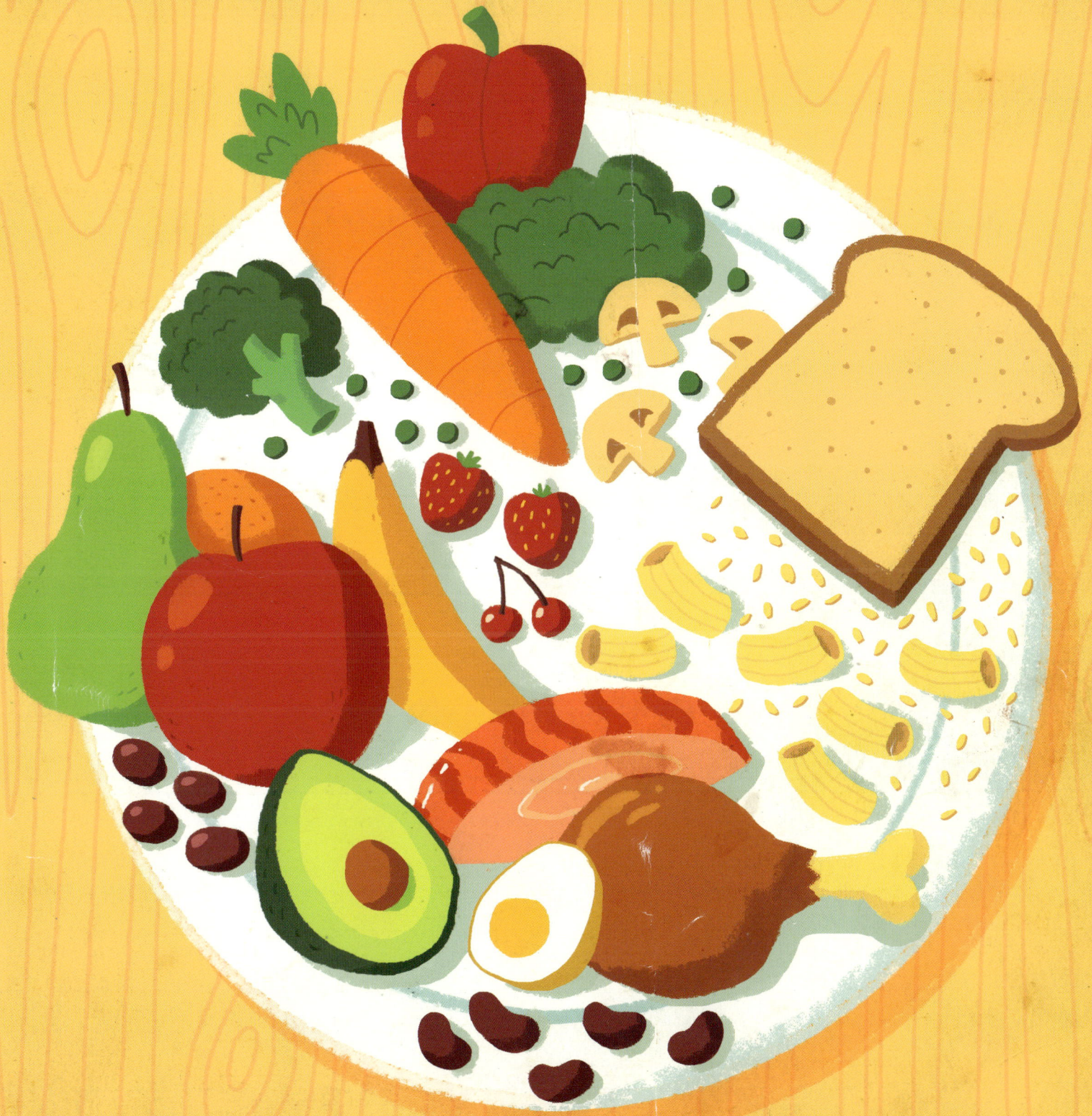

What should I drink?

Did you know that more than half of your body is made of water? Your body needs water to work as it should and stay alive. Some of this water comes from the food you eat, but you also need to drink plenty of water every day to stay healthy. To get enough water, choose it over other drinks when you feel thirsty.

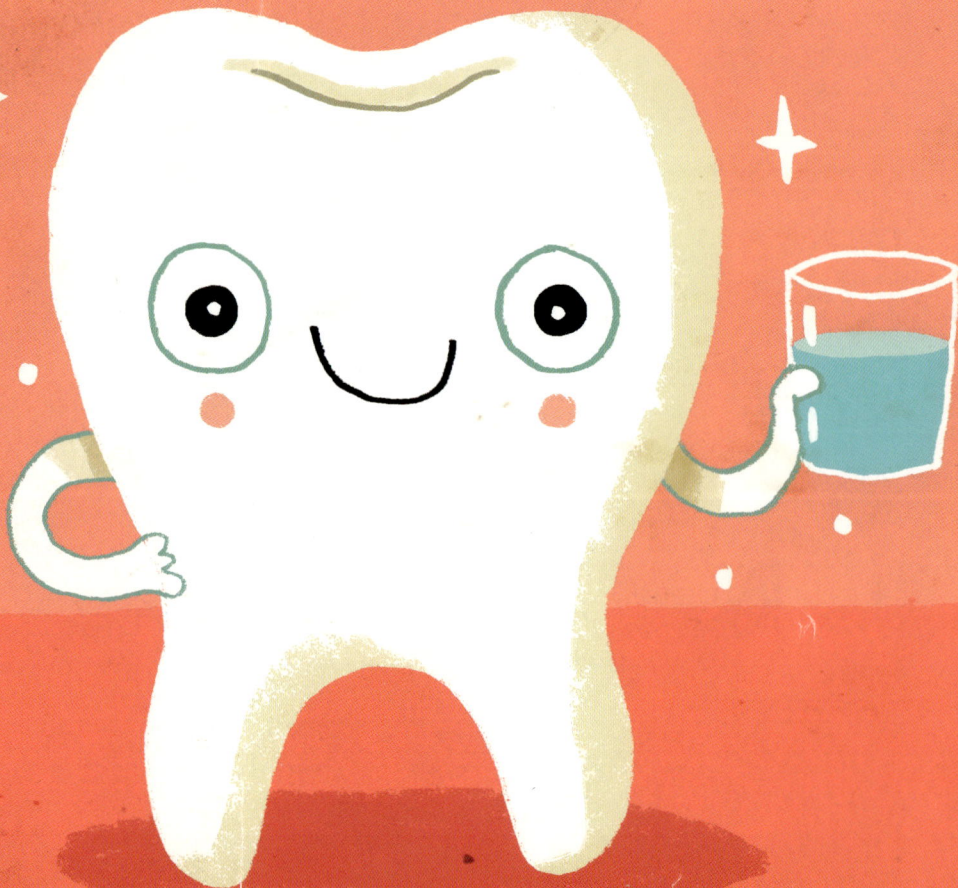

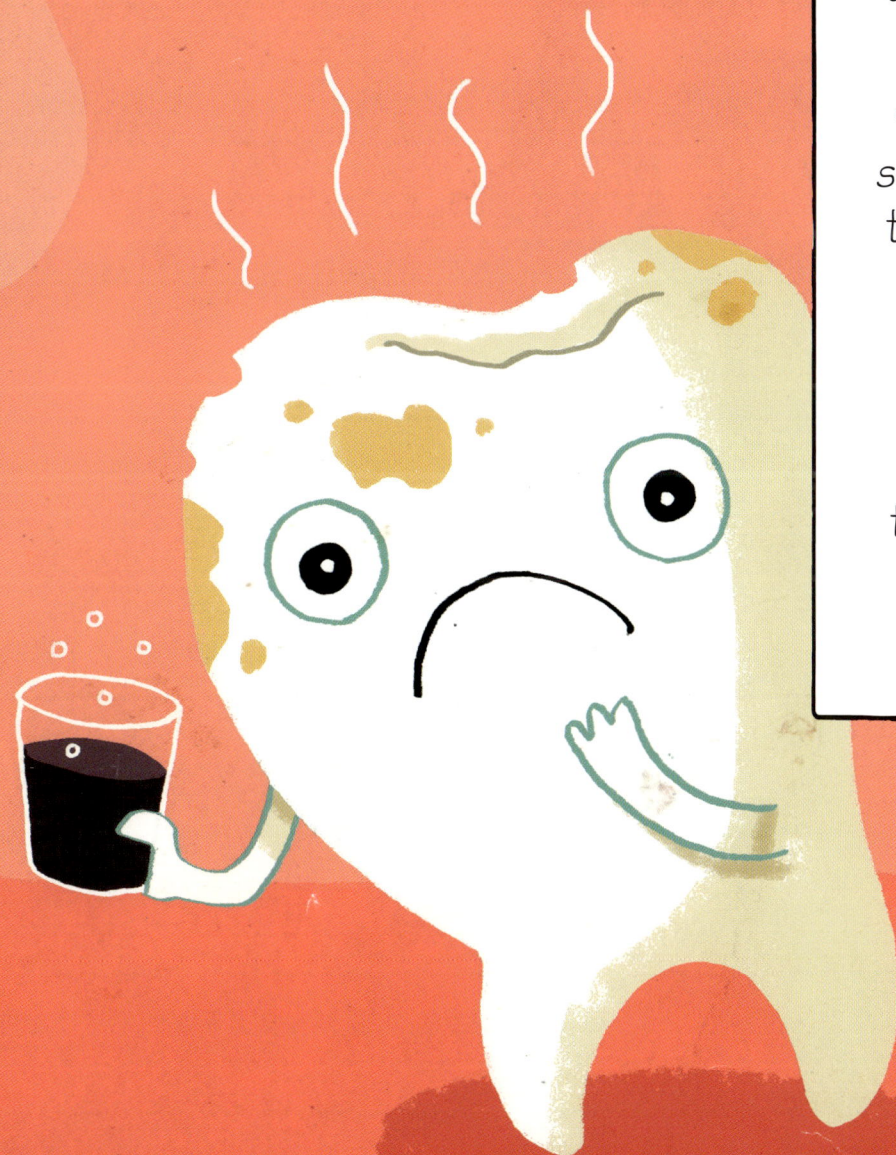

What can I do?

• Water is the best drink for you. Milk can also be a good choice because it is good for your bones.

• Drinks that have added sugar are not good for your teeth. These drinks include lemonade, pop, and even fruit juice.

• It's best to think of sweet drinks as special treats. They should not be a choice every day.

Treats

Treats are things like chocolate, ice cream, cookies, and chips. They are things many people really enjoy eating! However, treats don't have much goodness for our bodies. They don't give us a lot of energy or help our bones and teeth. Like sweet drinks, they can harm our teeth.

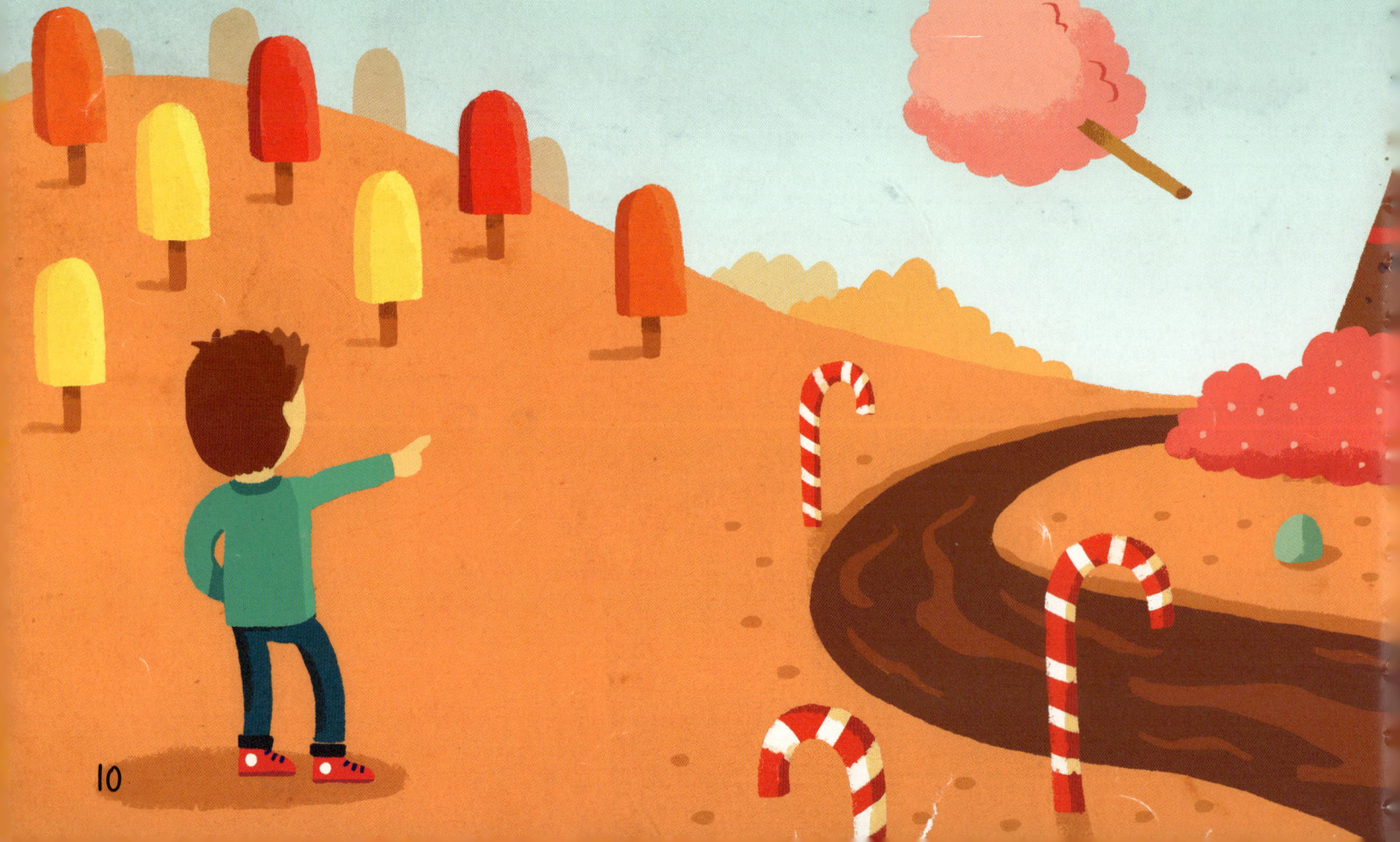

If you are hungry for something sweet,
try eating a piece of fruit instead!
It is OK to enjoy treats sometimes,
but not every day.

Be active

Remember the bones, muscles, and organs you depend on? They need exercise to stay healthy. Exercise is anything that gets you moving. To stay active, exercise for around 60 minutes every day.

What can I do?

Here are some good ways to get exercise. Which is your favorite?

- Swimming
- Walking
- Riding a bike
- Running
- Dancing
- Playing sports

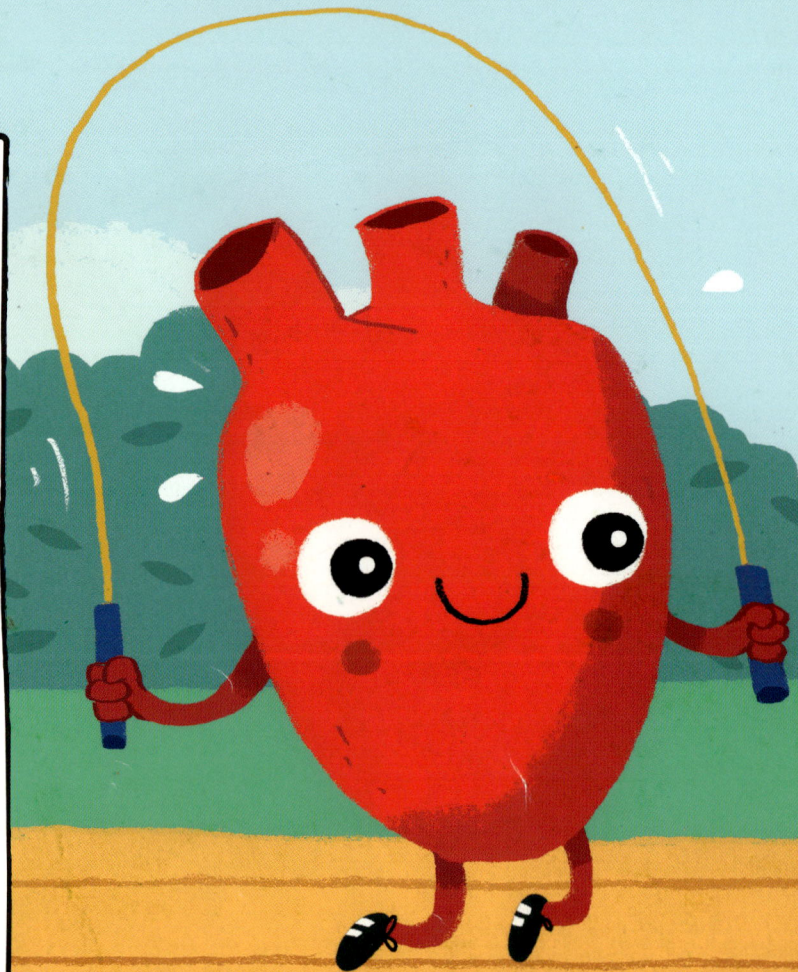

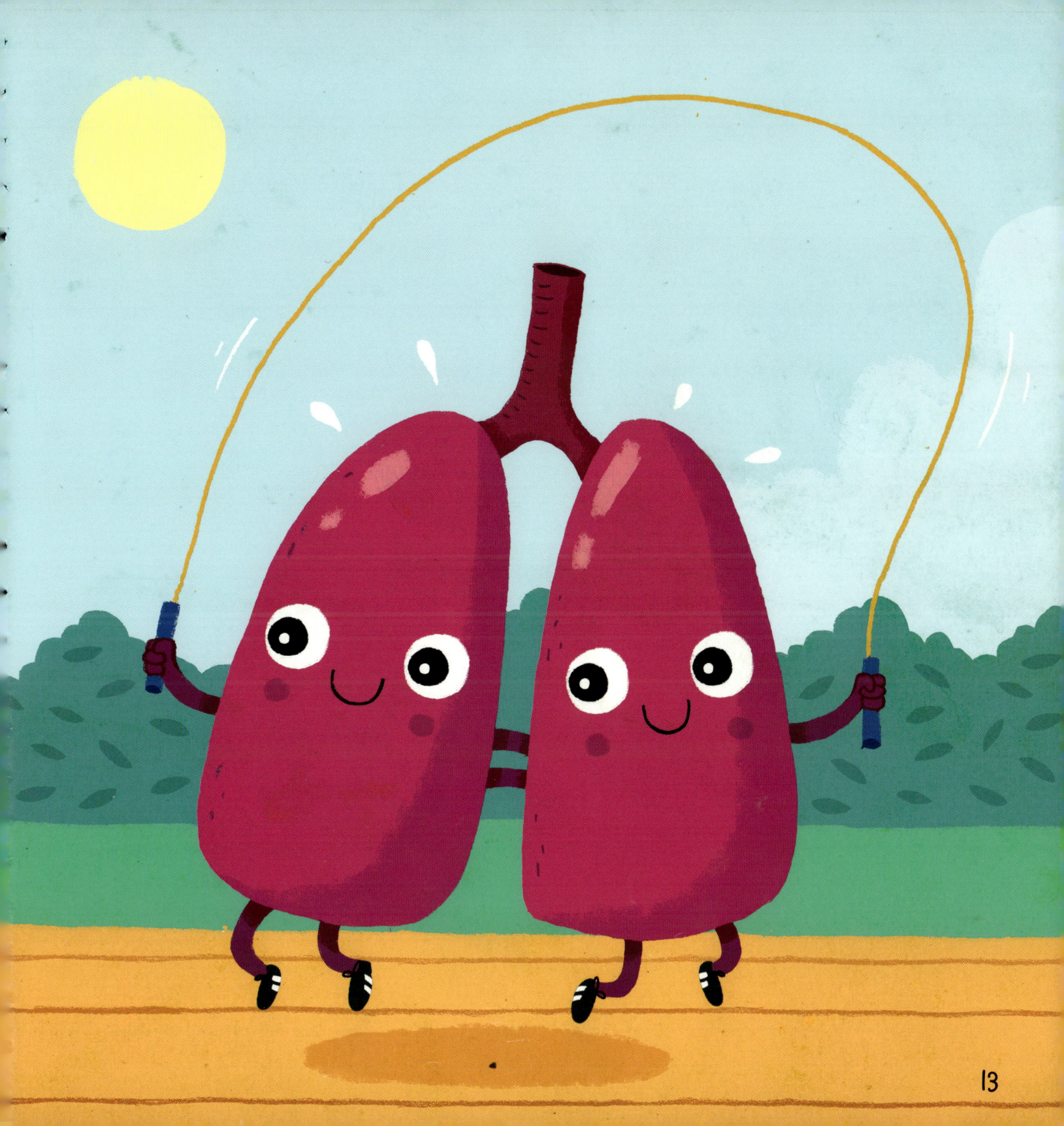

Keep clean

Do you like taking baths, or is it more fun to play in the mud? One way to stay healthy is to keep your body clean!

Taking a bath or shower two or three times a week is important. You should wash your hair and body with soap. When you're clean, use a towel to dry off and put on clean clothes.

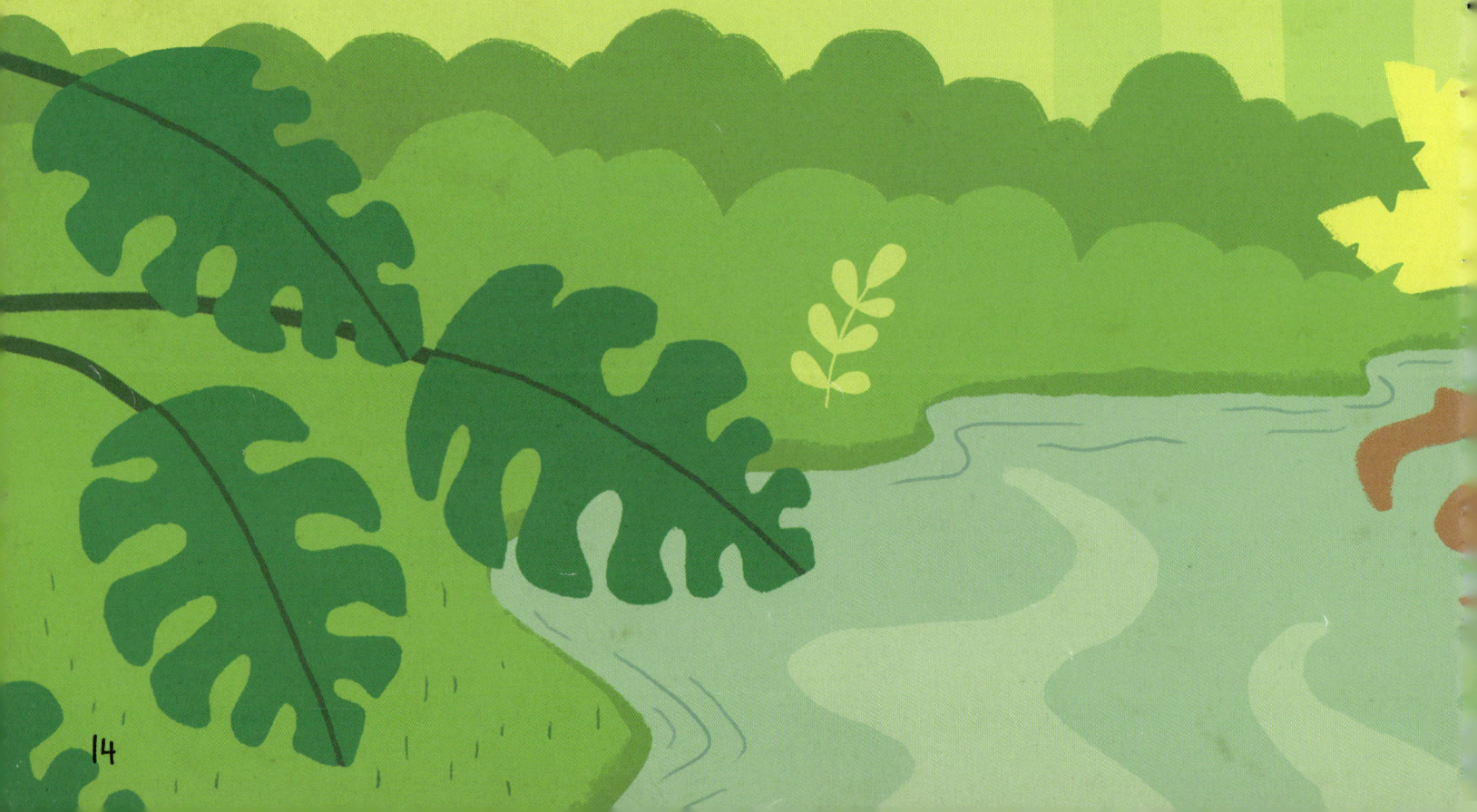

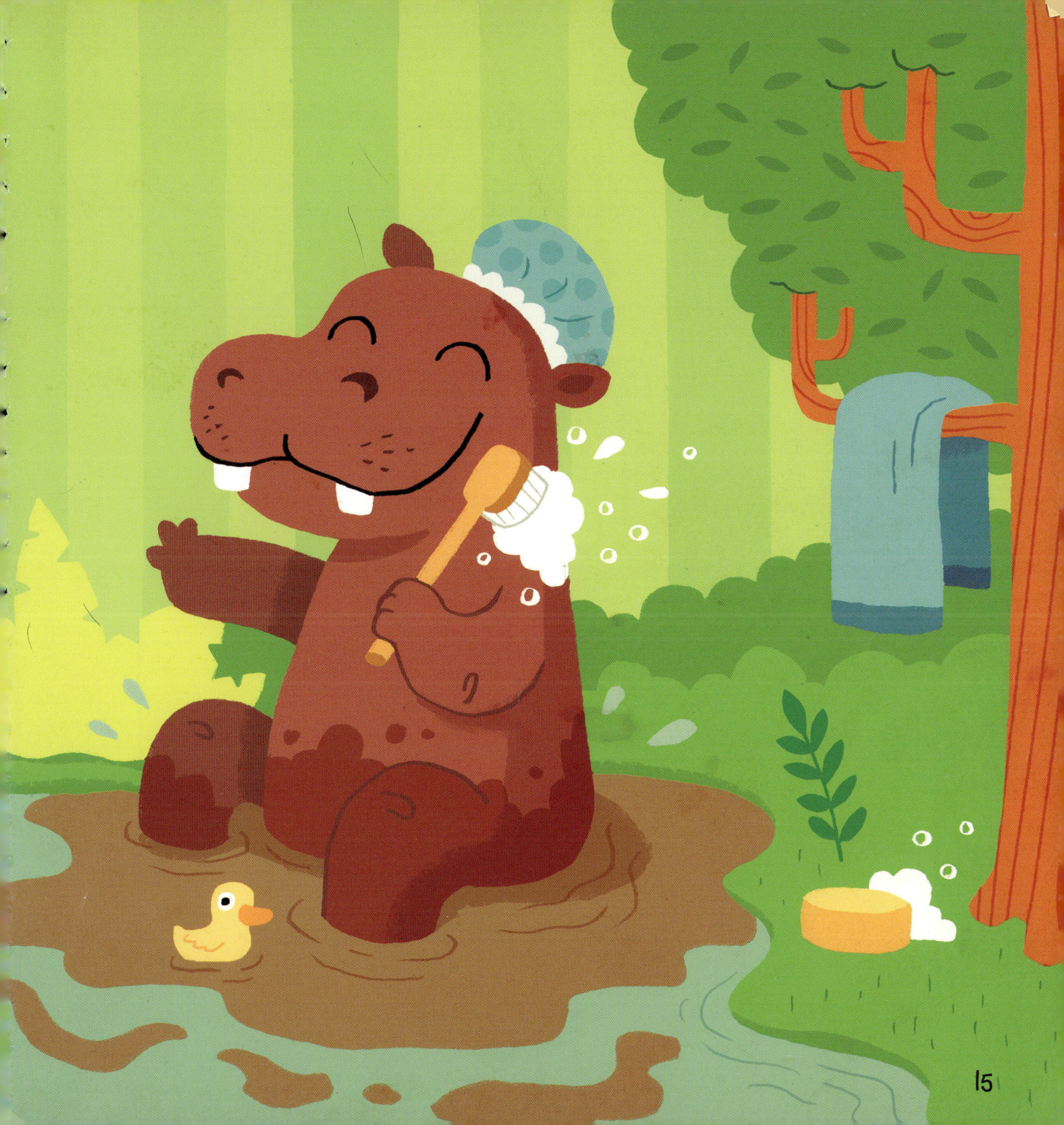

Wash your hands

Think about how much you use your hands! You touch many surfaces and objects all day. Then, you might touch your eyes, nose, and mouth. Any **germs** on your hands will then enter your body. That is why it is so important to keep your hands clean. You should always wash your hands after you use the toilet and before you eat. Try not to touch your face if you have not washed your hands.

What can I do?

Here's how to wash your hands:

1. Use warm water and soap.

2. Rub your hands together and create suds. Make sure the suds clean all parts of your hands—even between your fingers.

3. Don't rush! Try singing the "Happy Birthday" song in your head twice—that's about how long it should take.

4. Dry your hands with a clean towel.

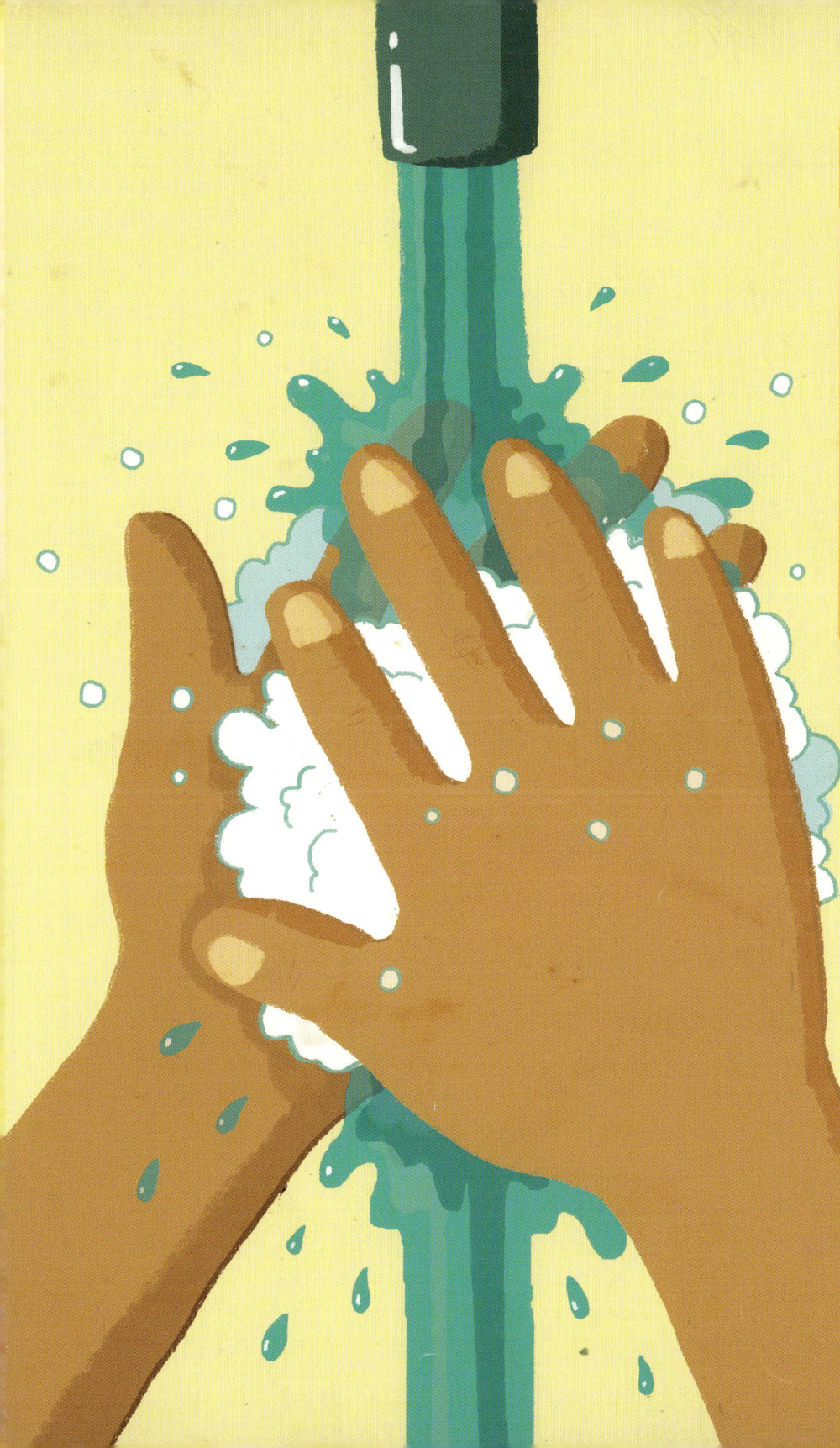

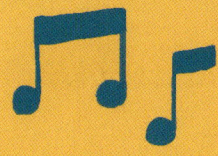

Happy
birthday
to you...

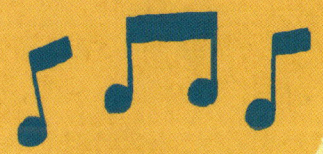

Take care of your teeth

Think about how useful your teeth are. They help you to chew your food. They also help you to talk and smile! Everyone has only two sets of teeth in their lives. Your baby teeth start to fall out when you are around six years old. By the time you are around 14, you should have all your adult teeth. They have to last for the rest of your life! Teeth that aren't looked after start to break down. They can get holes in them called cavities. That's why it is very important to take care of your teeth.

What can I do?

- Brush your teeth at least twice a day with toothpaste.
- Make sure you brush every part of each tooth. Brush teeth in the front and back of your mouth equally.
- Use a toothbrush with soft bristles and ask your parent or caregiver for a new one every three months.
- Floss your teeth once a day to get rid of food that your toothbrush missed.
- Your parent or caregiver should take you to visit the dentist twice a year to check that your teeth are healthy. The dentist will check for signs of cavities.

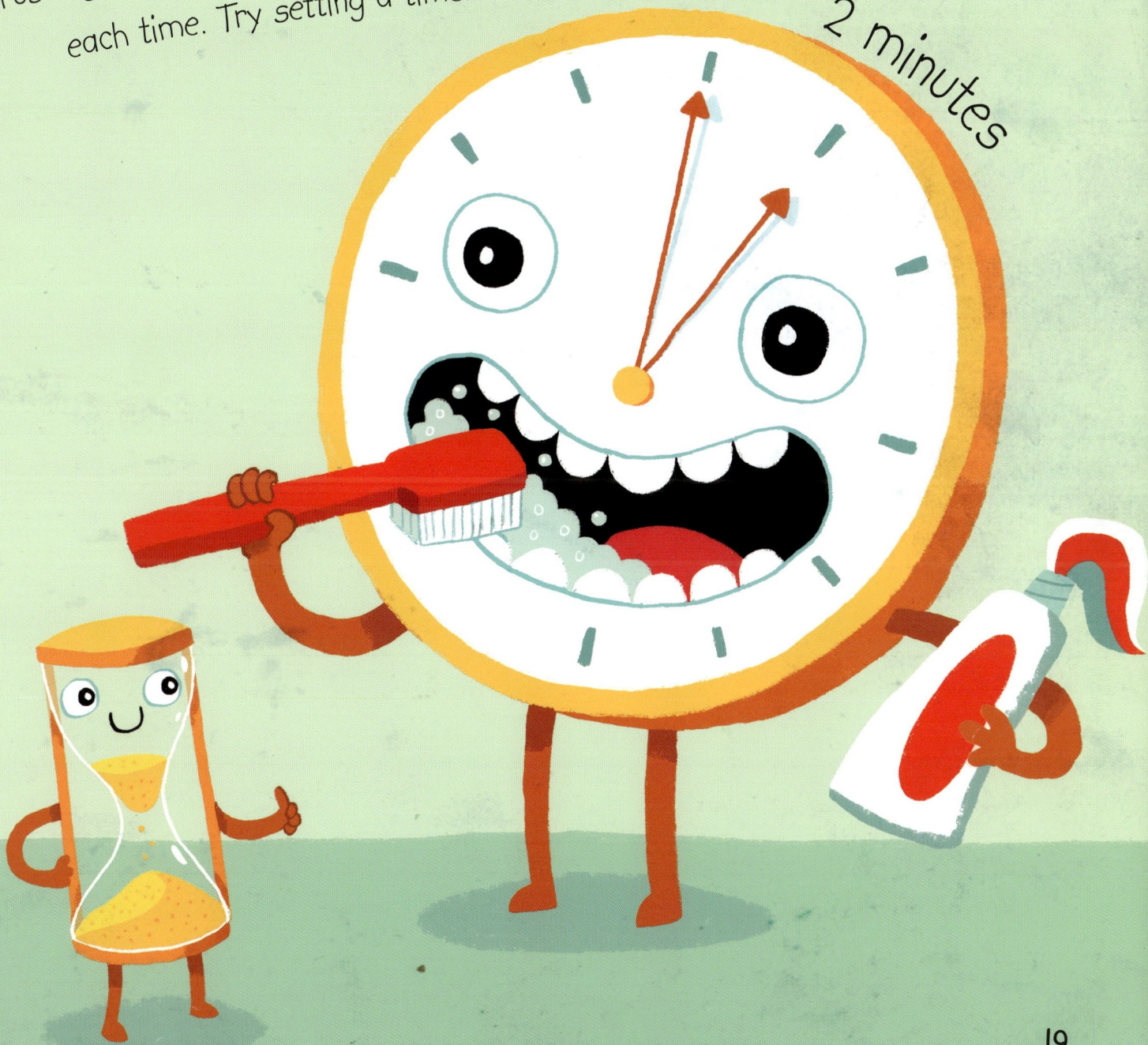

Brushing should take around two minutes each time. Try setting a timer!

2 minutes

The skin you're in

Your skin is an organ that covers all of your body. It does many jobs. It protects your inner body. It keeps germs out and helps your body stay the right **temperature**. It also **senses** how things feel. One of the ways to keep your skin healthy is to drink plenty of water.

You also need to be careful in the Sun. On sunny days you need to wear sunscreen to protect your skin.

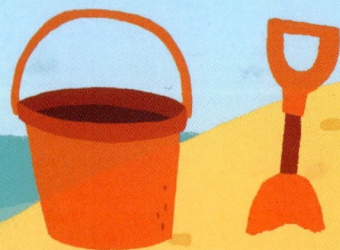

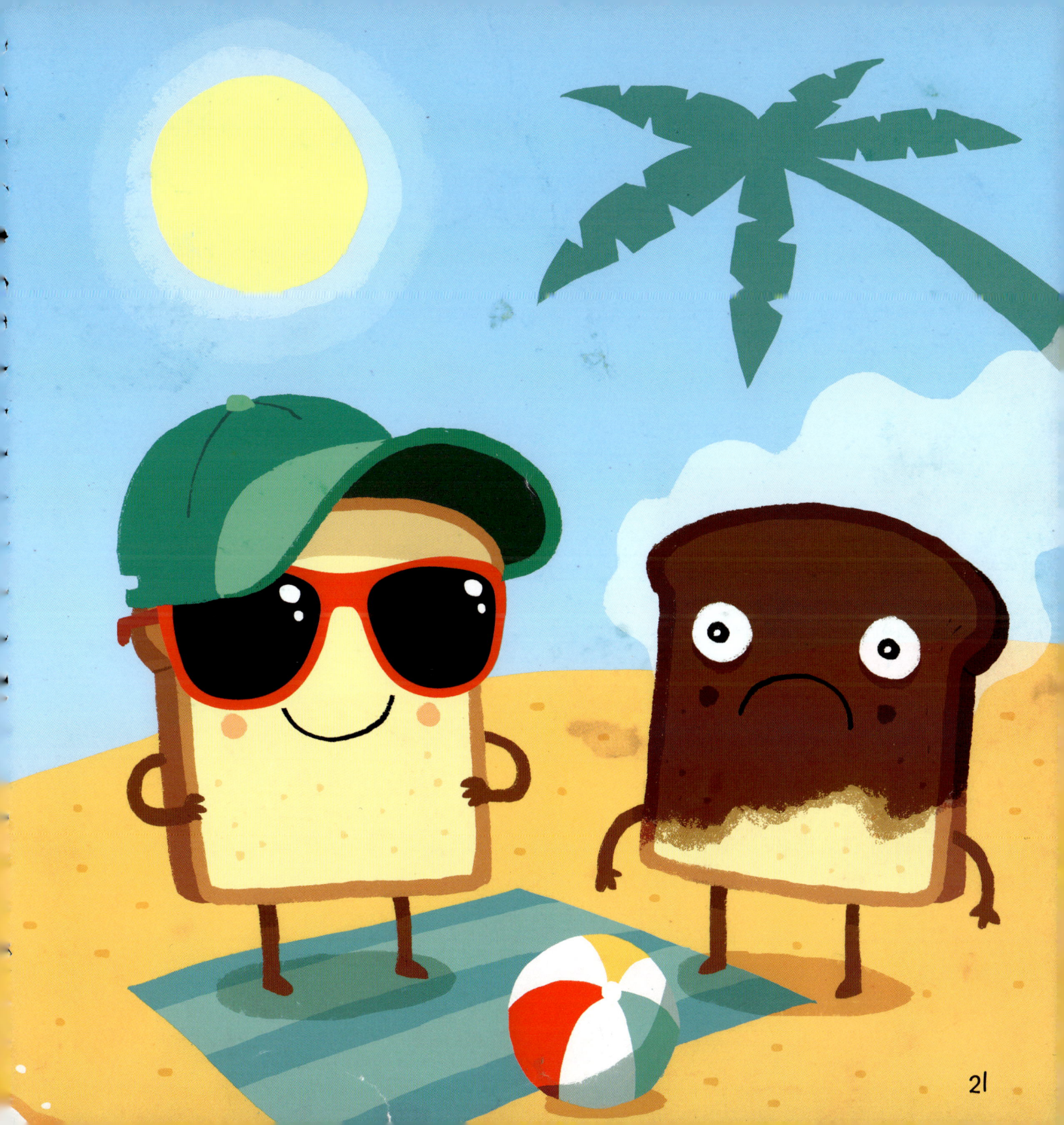

A good sleep

Did you know that children need more sleep than adults? Children are growing bigger and stronger and their brains are changing. They need a lot of rest to grow and change in a healthy way.

What can I do?

If you're struggling to get enough sleep, here are some tips:

- Daily exercise will help you feel more tired.

- Try setting an earlier bedtime.

- Try to "wind down" before you sleep. Do something that makes you feel calm, such as having a bath or reading a book.

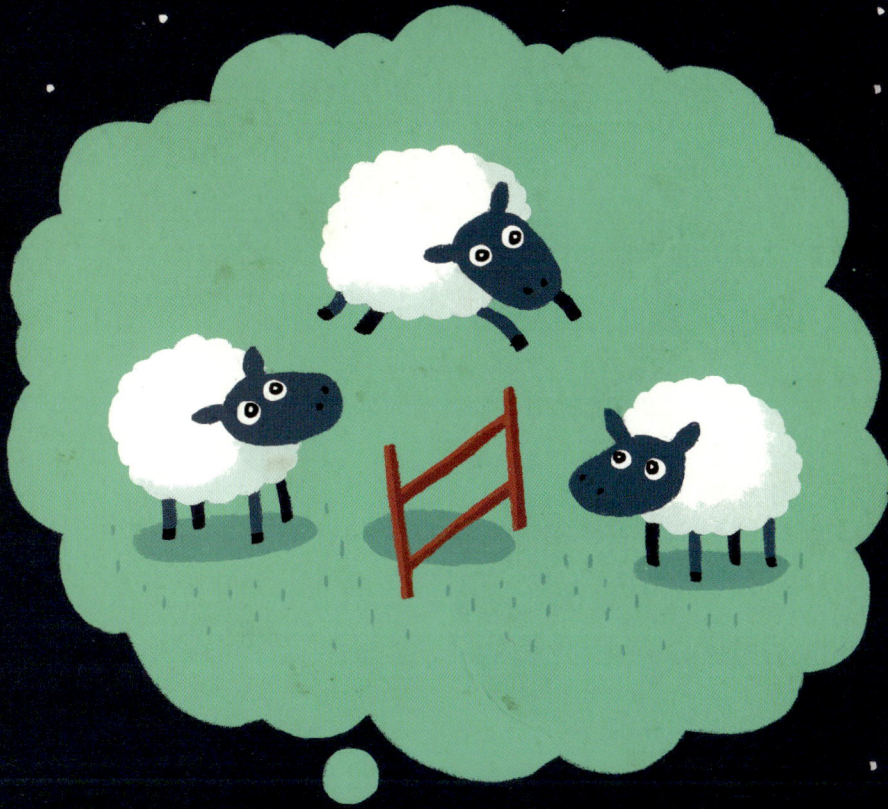
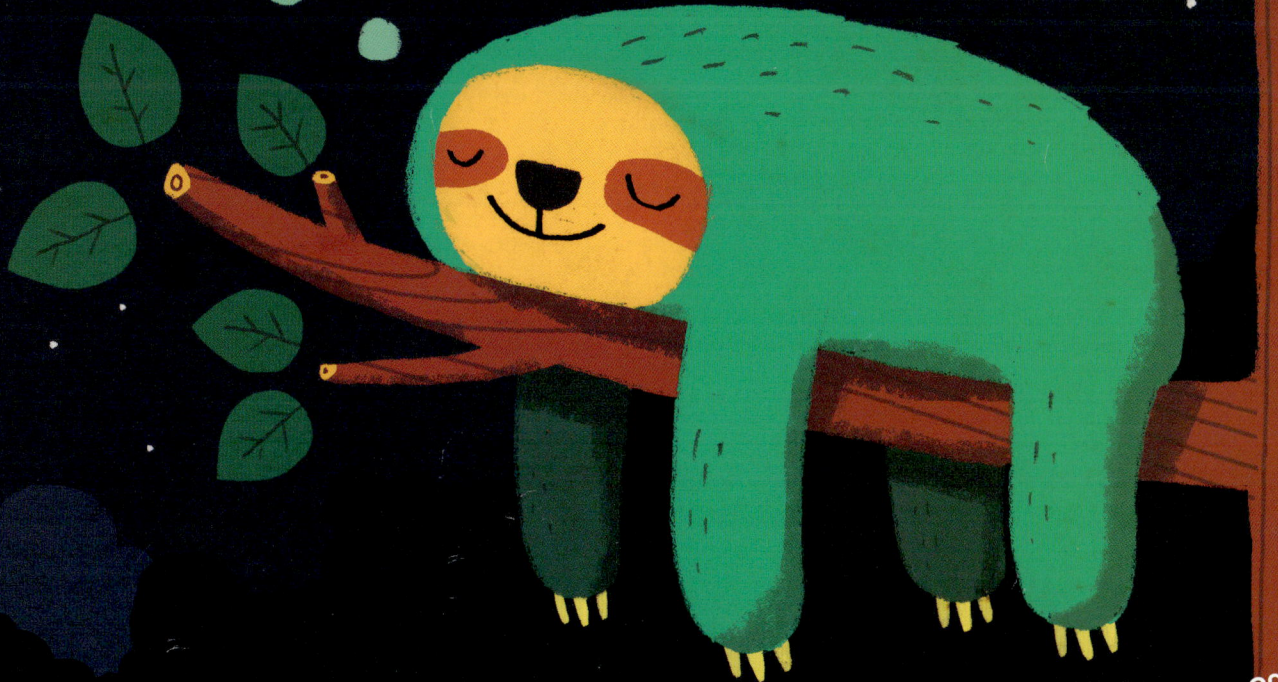

Feeling sick

Everyone gets sick sometimes. Coughs and colds are easy to catch from others. We might also catch **bugs** that make us ache or need to go to the bathroom more often. All of these bugs are too small to see.

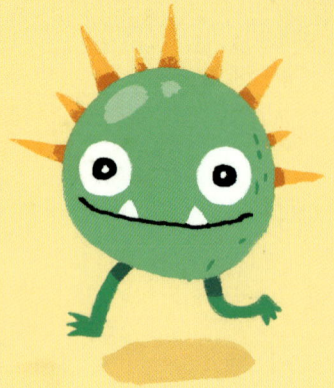

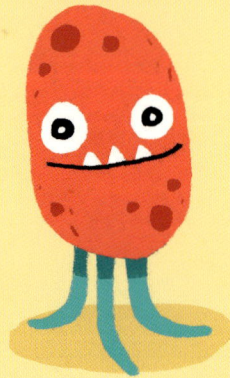

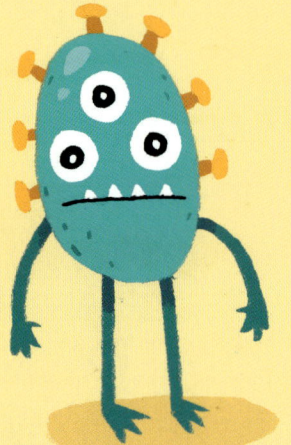

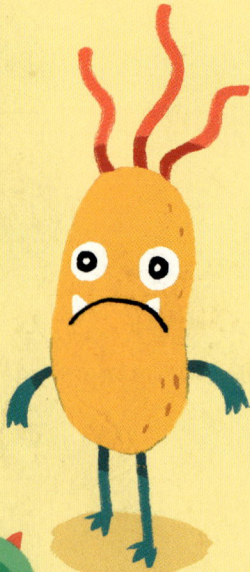

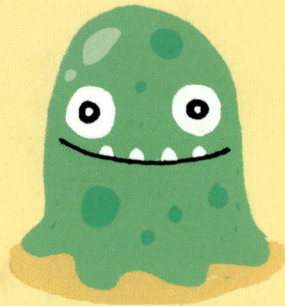

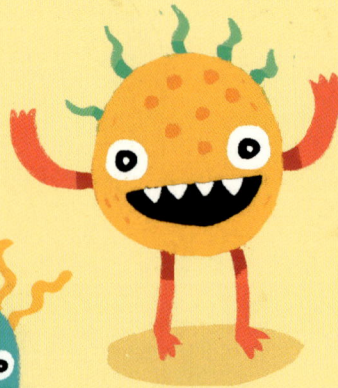

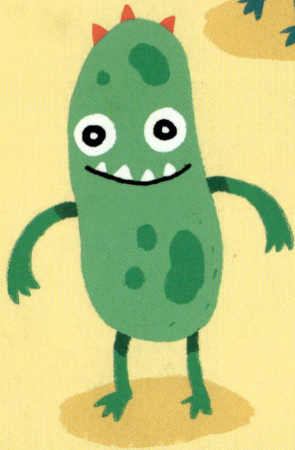

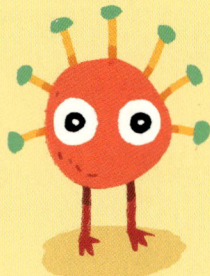

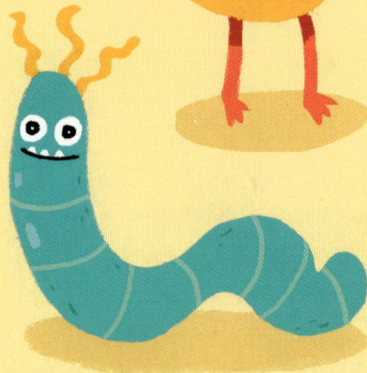

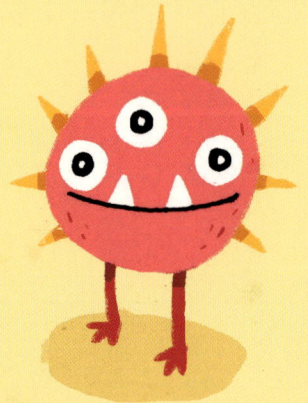

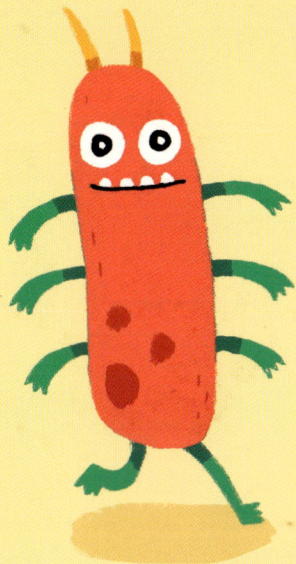

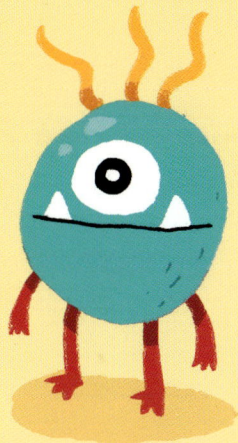

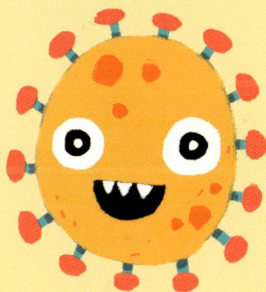

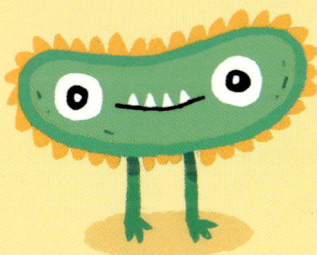

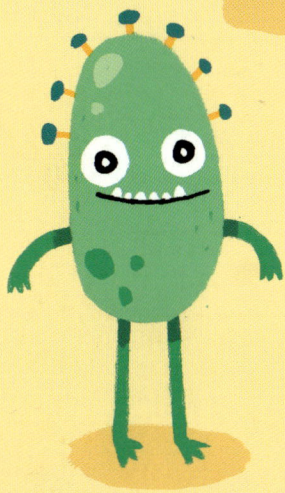

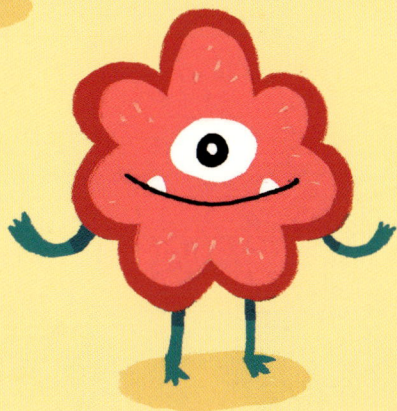

What can I do?

If you get sick:

• Cover your mouth and nose with a tissue when you cough or sneeze.

• Wash your hands often and well—follow the tips on page 16.

• Get plenty of sleep. Your body needs rest to fight the bug.

The good news is that actions such as washing your hands and getting a good night's sleep can help you avoid bugs most of the time. When your body is healthy, it can fight bugs well.

Visiting the doctor

Sometimes you may have to visit the doctor when you are sick. The doctor will check how the illness is making you feel and how your body is fighting it. Seeing a doctor is no reason to be worried. They will help you get better.

The doctor may give you medicine to help you get better.
It is very important to only take medicine given
to you by your doctor, parent, or caregiver.
Hopefully, you will feel better in no time!

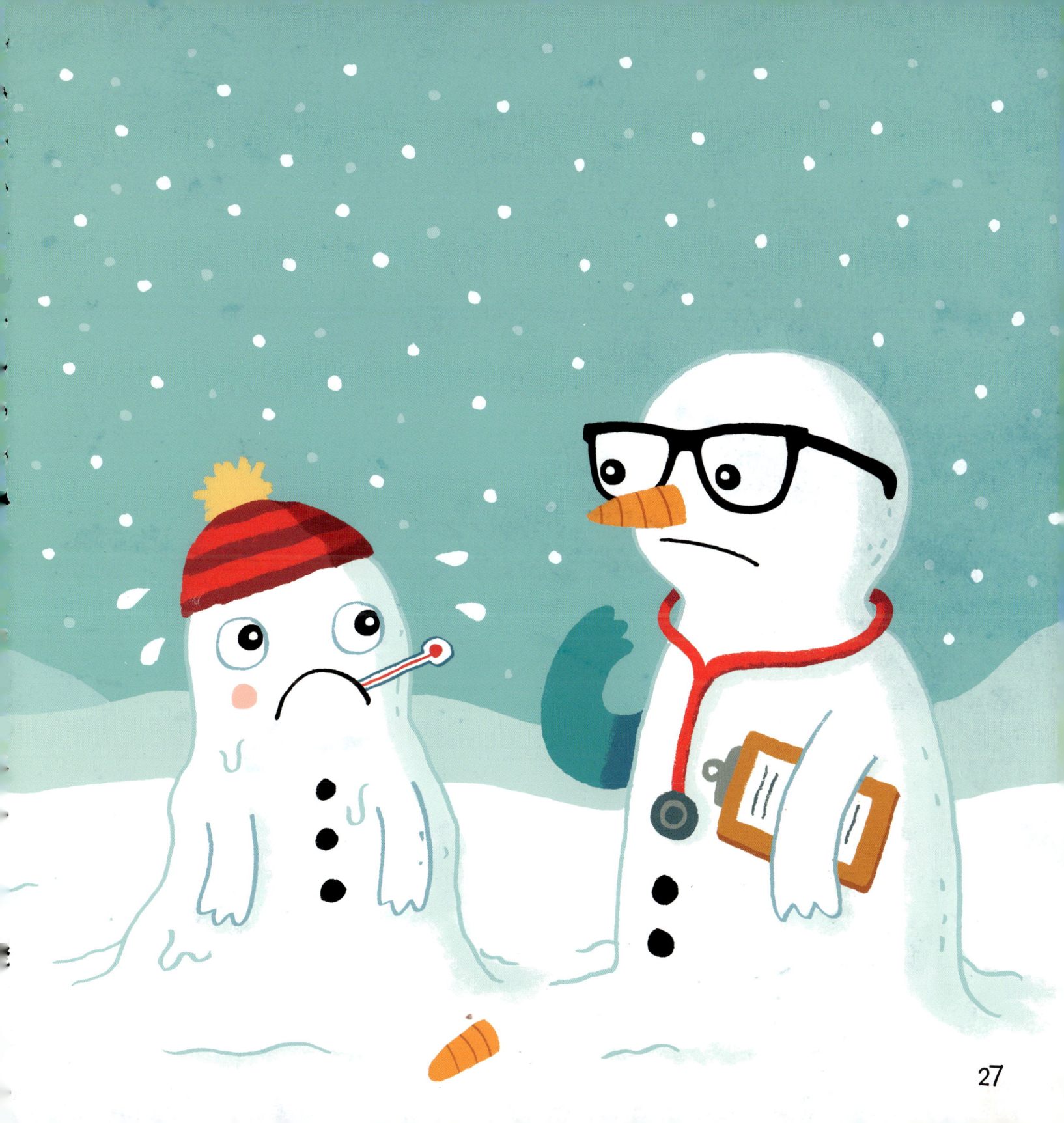

Your body for life

You only have one body all of your life, so it's up to you to look after it!

Did you know that your brain and body are connected? Thinking positively can actually help your body stay healthy.

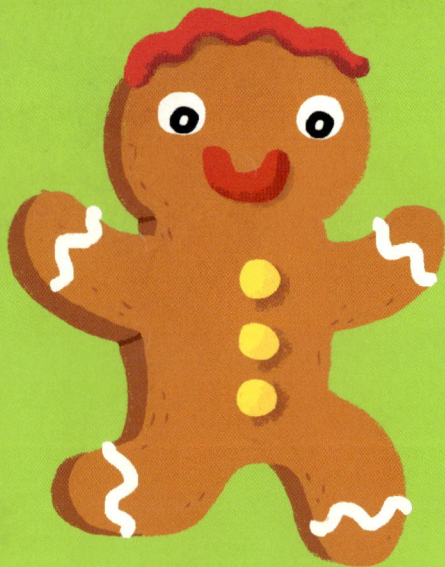

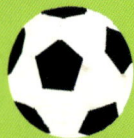

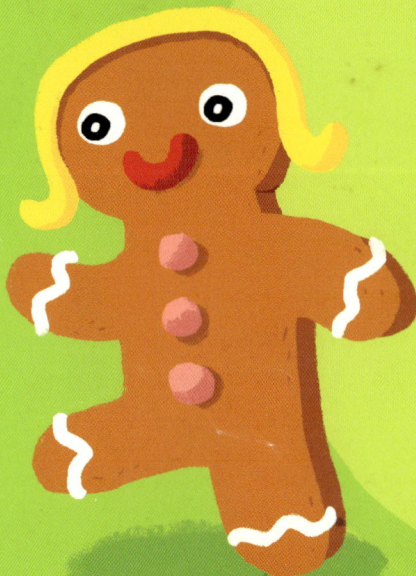

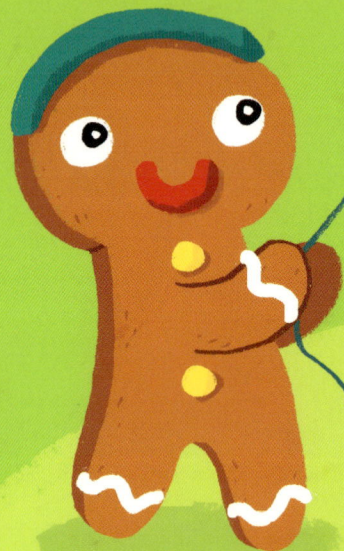

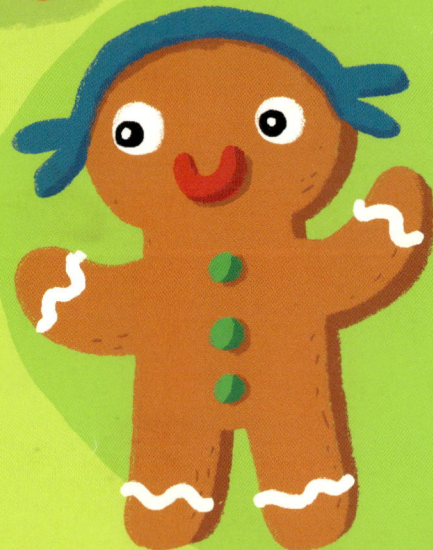

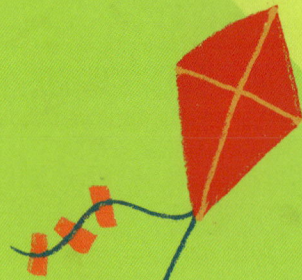

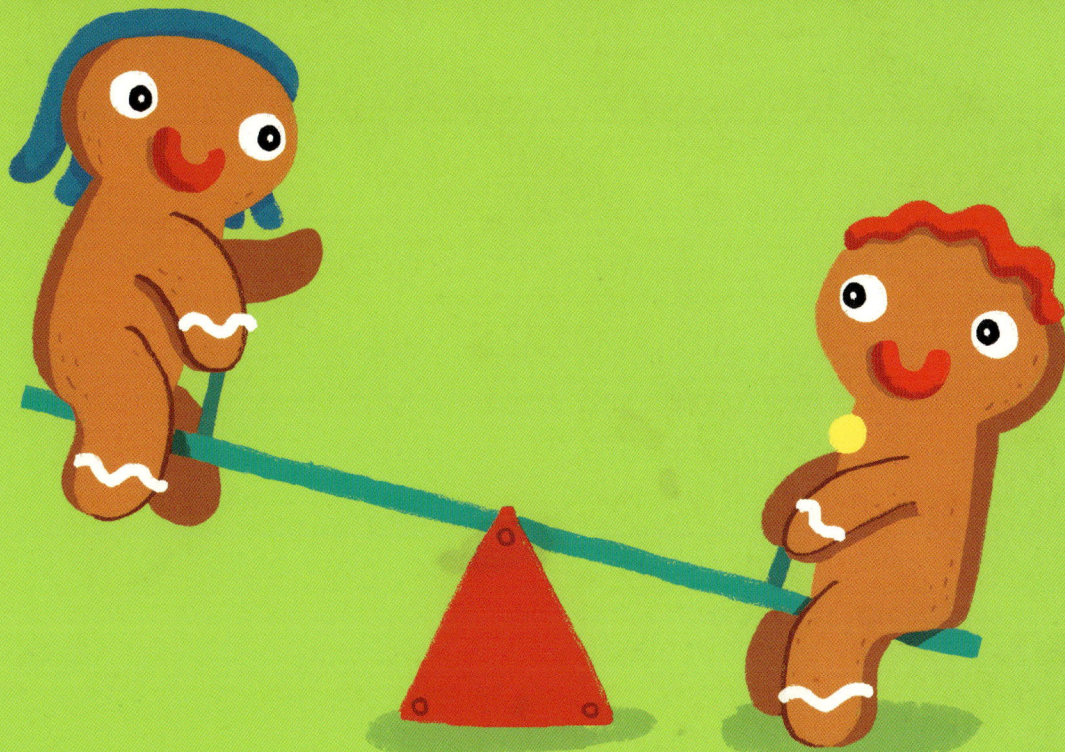

It is normal to have negative thoughts sometimes. This might happen when you notice others have different abilities than you. Maybe your friends are better at playing soccer, for example. But you can think positively by paying attention to your own abilities. You can practice skills, stay healthy, and notice when you get stronger or better at something.

Remember...

Drink plenty
of water.

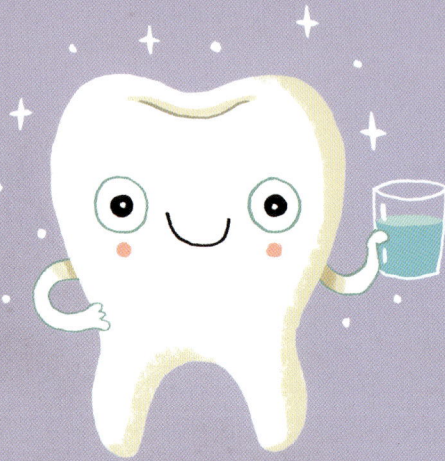

Eat many
different healthy
foods.

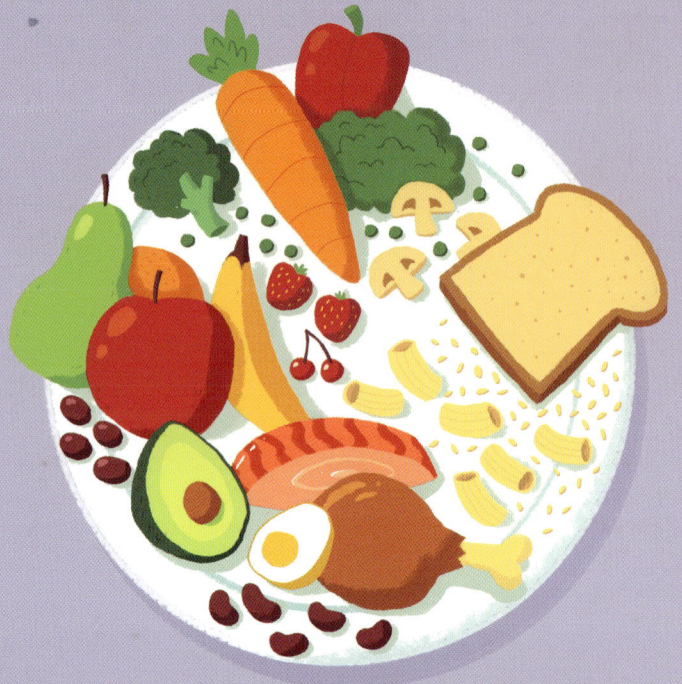

Getting enough sleep
is important.

Clean your teeth
by brushing twice
and flossing once
per day.

Wash your hands
before you eat
and after you
have been to
the bathroom.

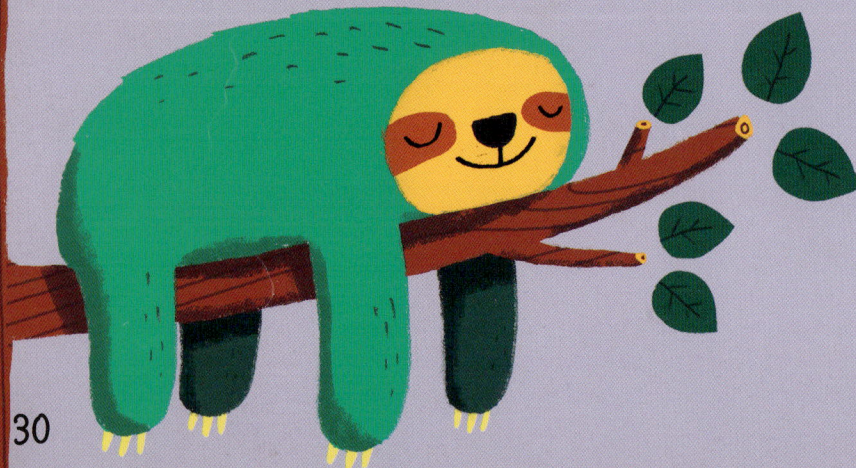

Exercise keeps your
bones, muscles, and
organs such as your heart
and lungs healthy.

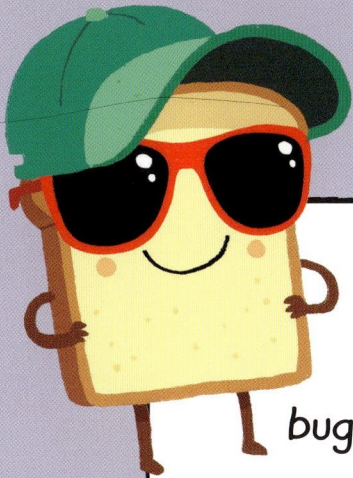

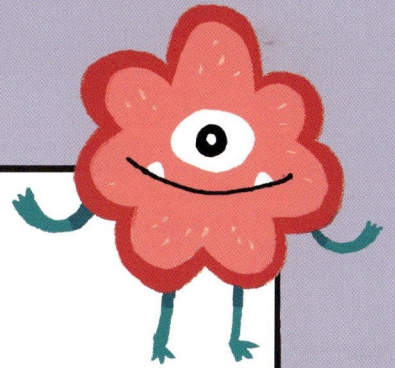

Words to Know

bug   An illness that comes from tiny bacteria or a virus

energy   The power to move and do work

germs   Living things, which are too small to see, that cause diseases

muscles   Parts of the body that you use to move your bones

organs   Parts of the body that have certain purposes

senses   The body's abilities such as taste, touch, sight, smell, and hearing

temperature   A measure of how hot or cool something is

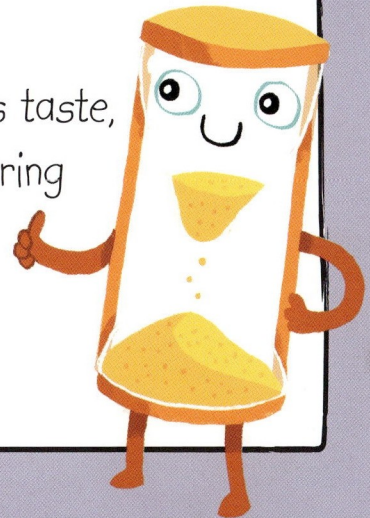

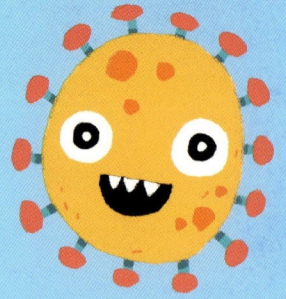

Index